Adult Coloring Books

An Introduction To The Healing Powers Of Coloring Mandala Pages

Lamees A.

CONTENTS

CHAPTER 1
WHAT EXACTLY IS A MANDALA?

I awaken to the power of the mandala,
A sacred circle of light and energy,
A pathway to center—to my center and to the universal All,
A channel for healing body, mind, and spirit.

Mandalas are more often than not, associated with the Tibetan form of Buddhism. Thanks to a lot of celebrity interest in the Tibetan cause and the Dalai Lama, there has been a resurgence of interest in this wonderful practice of creating intricate circular patterns. But what exactly is a mandala? Most people would be surprised to learn that mandalas have been in existence since the beginning of time. In fact, their beauty surrounds and envelops us, without us being aware of it.

A mandala, in essence, is a sacred circle. The history of the word itself lies in the Sanskrit language, and the term mandala loosely describes a "circle" or "center." A mandala is actually a simple geometric shape without a beginning or an end. That is why it is often in the shape of a circle, and within its confines, it possesses the power to bring about a state of relaxation, balance the bodily energies, lead to an enhancement of creative prowess, and cause a healing of body and mind.

The good news is that the incredible power and goodness obtainable from a mandala can be harnessed and channeled using mandala coloring pages. But first we need to understand what the mandala is, in all its intricacy.

The mandala is above all a symbol, as well as a representation of the core tenets of Hindu and Buddhist spiritualism and ritualism. Though these may sometimes be in the shape of squares and triangles rather than just circles, they will always have a concentric structure. There will be an inherent balancing of the various visual representations signifying balance, unity, and harmony. Each of the mandalas will represent a distinct and unique concept. The ultimate aim of all mandalas is to bring about cosmic and psychic order. It therefore becomes a sign of our connection with infinity, which goes beyond our mere physical body and consciousness. Mandalas are often of spiritual importance to a specific person or group of people.

Though the Hindus pioneered in the use of mandalas as a spiritual tool, it is really the Buddhists who made the concept famous throughout the world. Mandalas are a tremendous aid in meditation, enabling the practitioner to achieve oneness with the universe. So effective are mandalas in creating this connection that all the major religions of the world have had some form of mandala-style visual imagery, though these may not have gone by the same name. In the Western world, for example, the Stonehenge monument, the ancient Roman amphitheaters, and the windows of medieval Gothic churches are examples of architecture trying to replicate a miniature cosmos.

In the Islamic world, too, mandala-like representation can be detected in the great tradition of using intricate geometric patterns of design in embellishing mosques, public buildings, and homes. These patterns were not created for decorative purposes only, but represented celestial models that existed both in the cosmos and within the souls of human beings.

The Navajo Indians of North America were long aware of the medicinal properties that were vested in mandalas, and would create their own out of sand.

Interestingly, mandalas also have a political meaning in the south and Southeast Asian context. Unlike the Western and Chinese definition of firmly demarcated external boundaries defining a nation, a mandala describes a more diffused pattern of power distribution where the center, rather than the boundaries, is of prime importance. This means that the center matters more than the extent of one's territory, thereby laying more stress on the local aspects of governance than building a mighty nation state. A mandala could contain a number of semi-autonomous power centers that form the sphere of influence of a regional central power. Personal relationships take precedence over official or even territorial associations in these types of mandala power centers. This appears almost absurd in today's times. But pause and think about it; is it really as bizarre as it sounds?

Mandalas can be put into three broad categories:

Mandalas That Instruct:

This is a highly symbolic mandala where every shape, line, or color highlights a specific aspect pertaining to religion or philosophy. Students hailing from diverse religious systems are instructed to create their own specific type of mandala that conforms to the prescribed pattern and method of construction.

This type of mandala is a condensation of everything that a student and practitioner of a particular system have learned. Essentially, a mandala of this type is really a colorful visual representation of the sum of the basic tenets of their doctrine, which the students are expected to know fully.

Mandalas That Heal:

These kinds of mandalas are simpler to make and are more guided by one's intuition than any rigid formula of construction. Its most basic purpose is to facilitate the process of meditation by creating the right conditions for calm and inner tranquility.

Sand Mandalas:

These are an integral part of Tibetan Buddhism, and are often created over a long period of time, with much labor and effort. Colored sand is used to create exquisite paintings, complete with symbols of religious significance. When ready, elaborate ceremonies are conducted atop these mandalas. The idea behind making these with sand is to bring home the fact that everything in life is transient and temporary, like structures built out of sand.

Lamees A.

CHAPTER 2
WHERE DO MANDALAS
COME FROM?

You don't have to look far to realize the abundance of circular patterns typifying the mandala in the very environment in which you breathe and live. Geometric patterns of the mandala are all around us, and touch every aspect of life. The life-giving sun, the very nuclei of the cells that make up our bodies, the orb of a raindrop, and the crystalline design of a snowflake encompass the sacred circle symbolized by a mandala. Mandalas have been a part of existence ever since the universe itself got created with a bang billions of years ago. It is this primeval origin that gives these patterns a primordial energy.

The ancient science of sacred geometry would have us believe that a mandala pattern is in fact created by the interlocking of spheres that form the grid of all ancient matter. We only need to look at the ancient origin of the concept of mandalas and their manifestations in so many indigenous practices in different corners of the world to realize how pervasive the influence of mandalas is since the time man became conscious of his environment on a cosmic level.

In that sense, the very beginnings of civilized behavior of mankind can be traced to its early recognition of the significance of mandalas. Man learned to acknowledge the power of the mandala by positive experiences that he could directly attribute to mandala patterns. That is why they began to appear everywhere across countries, cultures, continents, and religions, mostly independent of any outside influence.

Tibetan monks find the embodiment of all the fields of spiritual consciousness and enlightenment in the mandala. For the American Indians, the mandala is the medicine wheel that epitomizes sacred ceremonial spaces, and also the circle of life. Mandalas are revered in both Eastern and Western cultures as symbols of harmony, unity, wellbeing, and healing.

In truth, the mandala is all of these representations and more. The mandala encompasses all aspects of life—material as well as non-material. Our material life is defined by circles of our family, friends, and community. The non-material reality of life is represented by celestial circles embodied in the earth, the sun, and the moon. Come to think of it, religious structures such as temples, stupas, mosques, and churches usually have a building constructed around a center—the classic mandala.

The greatest and most profound of mandalas is the circle of life itself. If you have clarity of thought and purpose, you can experience an inner spiritual journey, even as you are enveloped by the outer world, much like a mandala presents an integrated view of the world. Once we become aware of this truth, we will change the way we view ourselves, the world that we inhabit, and above all, the very raison d'etre of our lives.

The famous psychiatrist Carl Jung was a big believer of the power of mandalas. He held that a mandala symbolized "a safe refuge of inner reconciliation and wholeness." He further maintained that a mandala was "a synthesis of distinctive elements in a unified scheme representing the basic nature of existence."

From a spiritual point of view, mandalas contain the secret code that unravels the mysteries of the universe. Working on creating a mandala or simply viewing one provides us with a glimpse into the makeup of the universe that intrinsically includes us. That is why we feel lighter and better after every interaction with a mandala, in whatever form that may be.

Come to think of it the sun, the raindrops, the petals of flowers, the egg encasing a little bird about to be born, the iris of the eyes through which we witness this dramatic world, and the very blood that courses through our veins uses circular pathways—the way of the mandala. Mandalas are really a cosmic key that take us above the mundane and make us one with what we really are—a vital part of a universe that is a throbbing, pulsating, and very much living force. Most times we are disconnected with this reality, and this takes away from our vitality and happiness. Reconnecting with mandalas reconnects us with that force.

We can imagine how powerful a tool the mandala is for self-realization, and if we were to access its power on a regular and sustained basis, we would be able to derive immense benefits from it. Mandalas are used to boost the power of meditation, which is the highest form of yoga, and is even known to help attain nirvana or salvation. People spend a fortune visiting state-of-the-art gyms, wellness centers, and spas that claim to use the latest cutting-edge technology to make them become physically fit. But physical and mental wellbeing go together. One without the other is incomplete and unbalanced. By choosing to color mandala pages, people can harmonize their minds.

These would help them grow more than their core body muscles. They would be able to grow their spiritual and mental muscles, which in turn would make them masters of their mind and body. Not only would that make them immune to diseases and stress, they would also be better equipped to achieve their material objectives.

Modern-day scientists don't pay much attention to

what mystics and philosophers have to say. This is not only unfortunate, but rather silly and naïve on their part. How can modern science—or what they believe is science by their definition—claim the right of being the only discipline that makes sense? This is highly ironic because some of the greatest scientists and mathematicians have been great philosophers as well—Bertrand Russel, is a good example of that.

"Many scientists think that philosophy has no place, so for me it's a sad time because the role of reflection, contemplation, meditation, self inquiry, insight, intuition, imagination, creativity, free will, is in a way not given any importance, which is the domain of philosophers."

~Deepak Chopra

Regardless of the fact that science has had to acknowledge the power of an ancient Eastern practice like the making of mandalas, they don't even begin to grasp the notion that mandalas are all about science. The human mind is a microcosm of the universe, and its capacity to perform is limitless. But this can't be achieved by studying at school or going to college and university. This operates at the level of intuition and experience. You gain knowledge not through immense effort, but through intuition. The knowledge itself leads to experience, and experience illuminates the path.

The movie *Kung Fu Panda* showcases this beautifully. The most unlikely of characters becomes the savior of the village, because within him lies the seed of greatness, which he himself does not realize. When the realization does come, it does not come by hard work or immense practice, but by intuitive realization of his destiny.

The mandala can take you to a world of immense intuitive power that can be highly transformative in your life, but only if you allow it.

"Personal transformation can and does have global effects. As we go, so goes the world, for the world is us. The revolution that will save the world is ultimately a personal one."
~Marianne Williamson

CHAPTER 3
HOW DO MANDALA COLORING PAGES ACTIVATE THE MANDALA'S HEALING POWERS?

Mandalas have been used to bring about a state of positivity and healing across cultures since the earliest times. There has to be some underlying reason for this amazing phenomenon. The clue lies in its design—a circular grid around a center point, which is the center of all infinite possibilities.

When you use your mandala coloring pages, you're expressing your desire for healing and wellness. You are making a pact with yourself to both acknowledge and utilize your limitless potential. It is like standing in front of the oceans of the world with all their waters at your disposal! While we are able to see the world around us to the extent that our physical faculties allow us to, mandalas can make you see inside you and realize how every part of you is connected to every part of the universe in the most profound way. This would be the epiphany of all epiphanies, and you would find peace, happiness, health, and everything else that you ever wanted for your asking. It would almost be akin to flicking a light switch and bathing a dark room in light.

There is so much that the human body and mind are capable of that it would astound most people. There is still no fully satisfactory explanation for how the massive blocks of stones needed to make the pyramids were transported across long distances so many thousands of years ago. It would be quite a task even in the twenty-first century. As Shakespeare once said, "There are more things in heaven and earth, Horatio, Than are dreamt of in your philosophy."

The mandala is a living and energetic pathway that can take you to the state of being you most desire. It may be anything—the desire for inner peace, to remove stress or merely your wish to create a breathtakingly beautiful mandala pattern. Whatever may be the reason behind your wanting to be involved with this process, mandala coloring pages can help you achieve just that. All you need to do is decide your objective and color the appropriate mandala pages, and you will see your deepest desires getting manifested. That is the long and short of it. The simple act of coloring the mandalas helps you in a number of ways.

• Helps you relax and meditate much better.
• Achieves a balance between body, mind, and spirit.

- Establishes a spiritual connection.
- Enhances your creative abilities.
- Improves your self-awareness.
- Makes you more expressive.
- Allows you to have a nice time coloring the pages alone or in the company of friends.

Lamees A.

CHAPTER 4
HOW DO YOU UNLOCK THE HEALING POWERS OF THE MANDALA?

By far the easiest and most convenient method of experiencing the healing power of the mandala is the use of mandala coloring pages. This is true for a number of reasons, not the least of which is the fact that the process of coloring is in itself a fun activity and quite therapeutic. It is a great outlet to give vent to our creativity as well. Anybody, regardless of their age, can be involved in mandala coloring.

When we are involved in creating a mandala, we are at the same time connecting with the immense intelligence that pervades every part of the universe. The trick is to relax, not overly exercise the brain, and open up to basic intuitive experiences while coloring the mandalas. The sheer power of the imagery that you will end up creating will become tools to make you grow as a person, and experience the endless possibilities that life holds for you.

Remember that great knowledge resides within the mandala. That is why the first thing a child will draw if given a pencil and a blank sheet of paper is a circle. The universe itself is not flat, and science tells us that light bends space. The mandala therefore represents the pattern of the universe. One of the most important things for people seriously interested in learning about mandalas is the fact that everyone eventually has to find their own specific mandala. A mandala has the power to let us have psychic visions, which makes us see a reality we don't normally experience in our day-to-day lives. Mandalas help us connect with forces of the universe we would not normally encounter in our everyday lives.

Modern inventions and so-called economic progress have caused a disruption in the progress of basic intuitive sciences like mandala creation. This has led to a spiritual imbalance and the science of mandala creation can help reverse this process. This is something that we need to profess loudly.

The world's free market economy model is driven by the growth model. There should be a certain percentage of economic growth every year or we end up facing recession. But how can this growth come endlessly when the resources are finite? How daft can one get? This is a one-way ticket to certain disaster.

There is a way of obtaining universal human

welfare using methods that don't ravage the earth.

Learning about mandalas is one of them. The universe is far more complex than we can perceive with our basic faculties. We do have hidden faculties that have the power and capacity to access these higher dimensions, and mandalas are the most significant tool to help us reach them. Among the most content people on earth are the inhabitants of the land-locked Himalayan kingdom of Bhutan. The Bhutanese people practice Tibetan Buddhism and understand that human happiness is far more valuable than material gain. That is why their government calculates the Gross National Happiness of the People (GHP) and not their Gross Domestic Product (GDP).

That is the kind of change of mind-set that there needs to be around the world. Mandalas—the most ancient of power sources that can transform the face of the earth—need to have a resurgence so that people in every nook and corner of the world realize its immense power.

It is not possible that everybody can understand and appreciate what the science of mandalas is all about. Neither will it be possible for people to understand the traditional ways of creating mandalas, or actually having the time or inclination to get involved in that manner. Coloring mandala pages, on the other hand, is the easiest thing in the world, and who knows? With time and practice, you may want to delve deeper into all that mandalas have to offer.

But even if we didn't, and restricted ourselves to

regularly coloring the mandala pages, we would obtain a host of benefits from the process—physical, mental, and spiritual.

There is every reason in the world for almost anybody to try their hand at coloring mandala pages and unlocking the healing powers of this process.

• Coloring mandala pages is an organic and intuitive process; there is no right or wrong way of going about it.

• There is no designated place where you must carry out this activity. Any place is good for you to start.

• Coloring is a fun process that makes you happy and gives you childlike joy.

• You can color at leisure and take as much time as you desire.

• There are no rigid rules to follow.

• Coloring is enjoyed by all, regardless of age.

• It encourages you to express yourself artistically.

• Coloring can be an enjoyable group activity.

• It is quite affordable.

• It helps you hone your intuitive skills.

CHAPTER 5
ARE YOU READY TO TAP INTO YOUR HEALING PATHWAYS THROUGH MANDALA COLORING PAGES?

Mandala coloring pages let you express your inner self and provide you a way of assessing where your life journey has carried you. There are so many suppressed and hidden thoughts and feelings that get expressed by the simple process of coloring the mandala pages and patterns. But above everything else, you are bringing to your life the healing powers of the sacred circle.

Don't believe for a moment that healing through mandala coloring pages is some mysterious fad that has become the flavor of the month. The stresses of modern living are now more acute than before, and conventional methods of healing do not even begin to address the root cause of what lies behind most ailments. Healing by the use of mandala coloring pages instinctively involves becoming whole, and thereby tackles the basic reasons behind people's ailments.

Our lifestyles are such that we make huge physical, mental, and emotional demands on ourselves all the time. This gets manifested in physical problems, and even has an impact on our relationships. However, the good news is that our bodies and minds have a tremendous capacity to heal, provided we create a conducive atmosphere of peace, quiet, and contentment. Now this is something the coloring of the mandala pages and patterns can most definitely bring you.

It will help heal at a deeply profound level, which we normally would not be able to attain any other way but by channeling the powers of mandalas. Our healing will be such that we will begin to feel in sync—not just with our own bodies, but with the whole cosmos surrounding us, enveloping us in a warm blanket of goodness and contentment.

Remember that mandalas are not mere drawings, but are sacred artworks that channel the energies of the cosmos—the same energies that flow within you and me—and using them put everything and everybody in a primeval harmony. The very colors that you use to decorate the mandala pages are infused with unique properties of their own.

The color white dispels ignorance and replaces it with purity and wisdom. Yellow removes the feeling of conceit and instead replaces it with kindness and compassion, while red helps get rid of attachment and fear and turns it into confidence and power. Similarly, green turns hatred into empathy, and blue turns anger into self-reflection and contemplation.

It is important to remember that the power of healing in mandalas was recognized by no less a person than Carl Jung, who was a psychiatrist used to treating people with mental illnesses. It is not surprising, therefore, to discover that mandalas have been extensively used as art therapy or as an aid to meditation. The use of mandalas helps treat people suffering from a variety of diseases, physical ailments and stress.

Mandalas are being taken very seriously by mainstream medicine. Clinical trials have begun to corroborate the value of these amazing circles of power in boosting the immune system, combating stress and depression, pain alleviation, lowering of blood pressure, and boosting the release of melatonin, the hormone that helps slow cell aging. Coloring of mandalas has the dual impact of art therapy and meditation, and is therefore that much more effective.

Mandalas are not so much pictures to look at as they are an invitation to enter fascinating worlds or realms. There is magic in the coloring of mandalas that takes an adult back to the childhood joy of coloring, as well as rejuvenates us spiritually. Coloring mandala pages is really akin to a relaxing and joyous journey into our inner self. People who have carried out the coloring of mandala pages report experiencing a sense of deep calm, contentment, and wellbeing. Considering the fact that it requires neither any training nor any practice, anyone can try their hand at it and experience its calming and soothing effects. Mandala coloring brings out the creative side in even the most seemingly non-artistic people.

Trying their hand at mandala coloring can be of particular use to children in coping with illness or emotional issues, and this is something that has been successfully tried at many hospitals. Similarly, it can be helpful to people trying to quit smoking, as coloring mandalas keeps the hands occupied. Even people recovering from life threatening illnesses like cancer can benefit from the exercise of coloring mandalas, and this again is something that has been put into practice in several hospitals.

Mandala coloring is clearly for everyone. But what it does need is advocacy. Not that it is not popular already, but given its sheer simplicity, negligible cost, and immense benefits, this is something that can be used to create a veritable health revolution. By popularizing the use of mandala coloring pages, whole nations can go a long way in addressing basic wellness issues, given the range of health benefits that accrue from this practice.

Creation Hymn

*Then was not non-existent nor existent: there was no realm
of air, no sky beyond it.
What covered in, and where? and what gave shelter? Was
water there, unfathomed depth of water?
Death was not then, nor was there aught immortal: no sign
was there, the day's and night's divider.
That One Thing, breathless, breathed by its own nature:
apart from it was nothing whatsoever.
Darkness there was: at first concealed in darkness this All
was indiscriminated chaos.
All that existed then was void and form less: by the great
power of Warmth was born that Unit.
Thereafter rose Desire in the beginning, Desire, the primal
seed and germ of Spirit.
Sages who searched with their heart's thought discovered the
existent's kinship in the non-existent.
Transversely was their severing line extended: what was above
it then, and what below it?
There were begetters, there were mighty forces, free action here
and energy up yonder
Who verily knows and who can here declare it, whence it was
born and whence comes this creation?
The Gods are later than this world's production. Who knows
then whence it first came into being?
He, the first origin of this creation, whether he formed it all or
did not form it,
Whose eye controls this world in highest heaven, he verily
knows it, or perhaps he knows not.*

The Rig Veda, Mandala 10, Hymn 129

Mandala coloring is an easy and astoundingly effective way of bringing about an immensely positive change in your life. So start coloring and enjoy it.

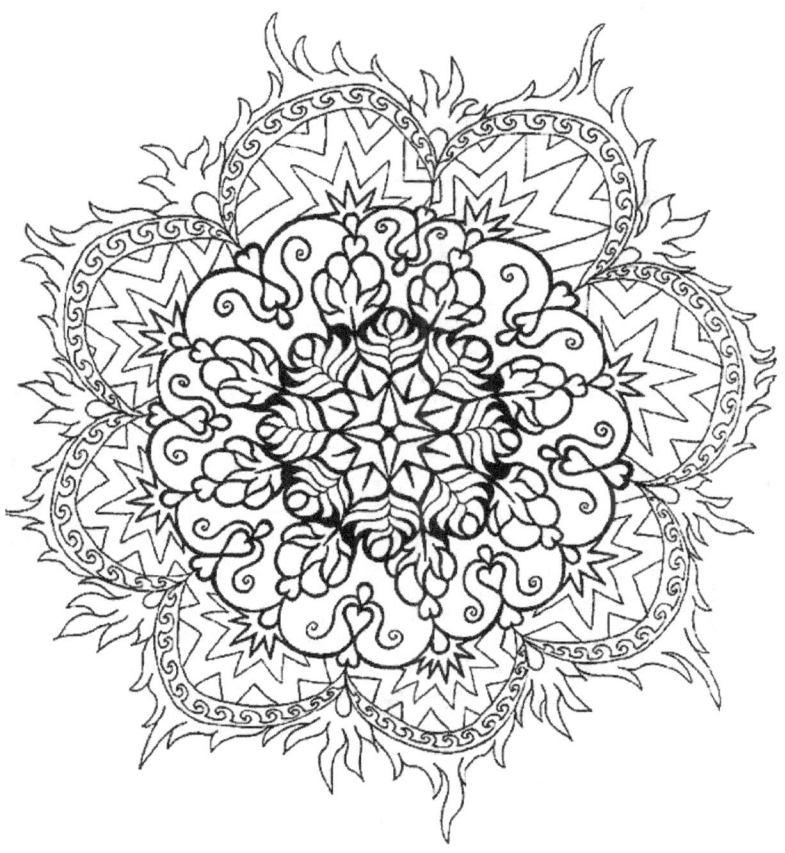

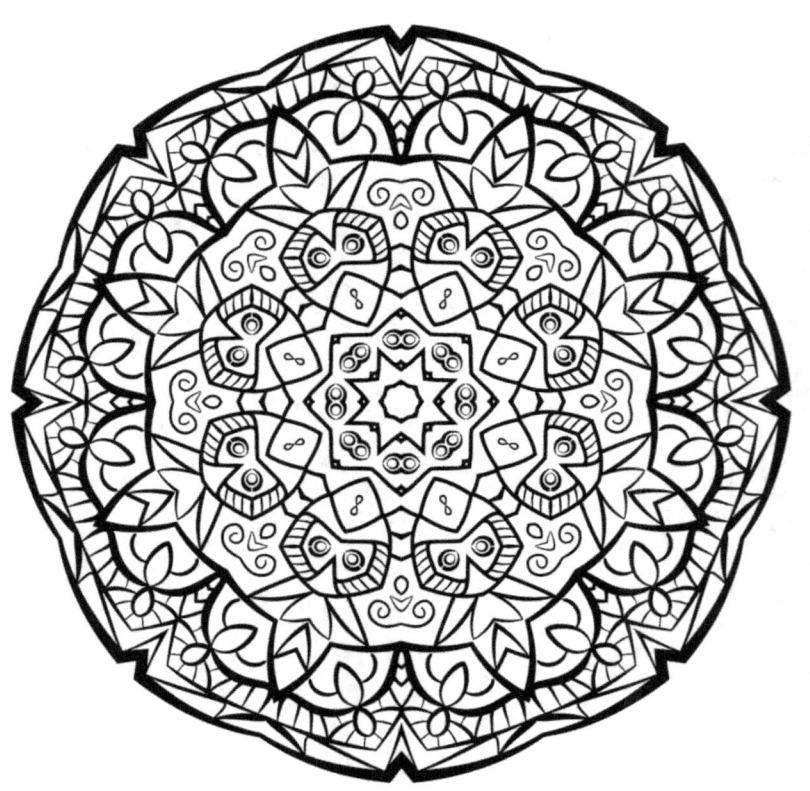

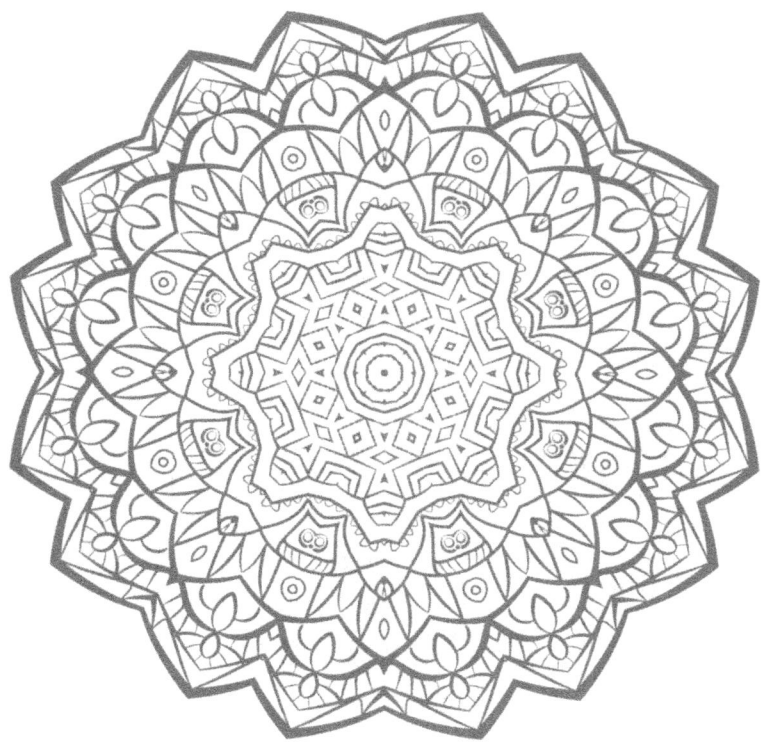

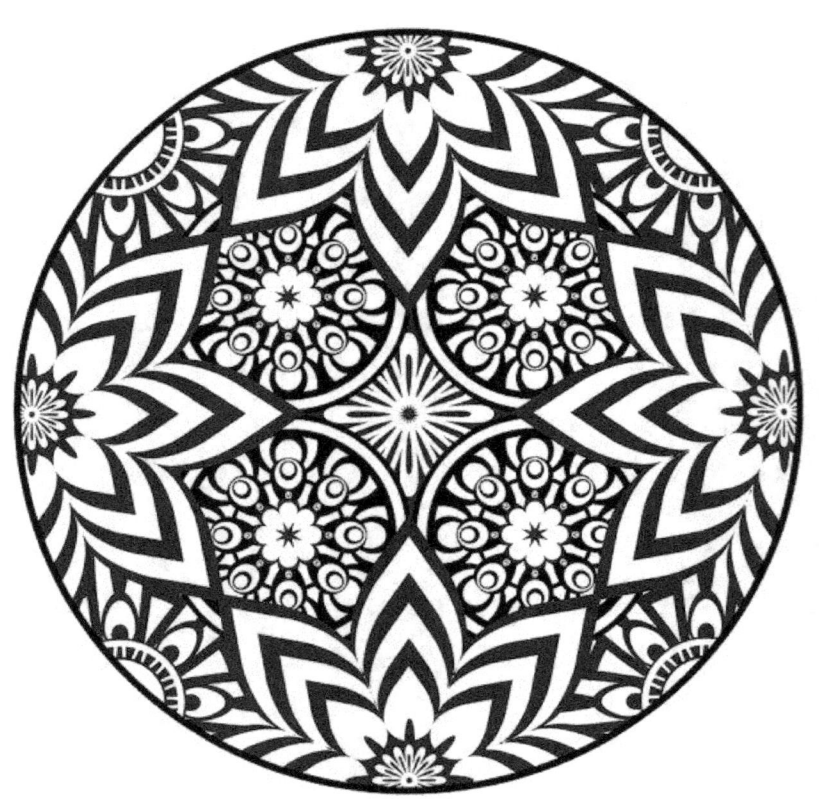

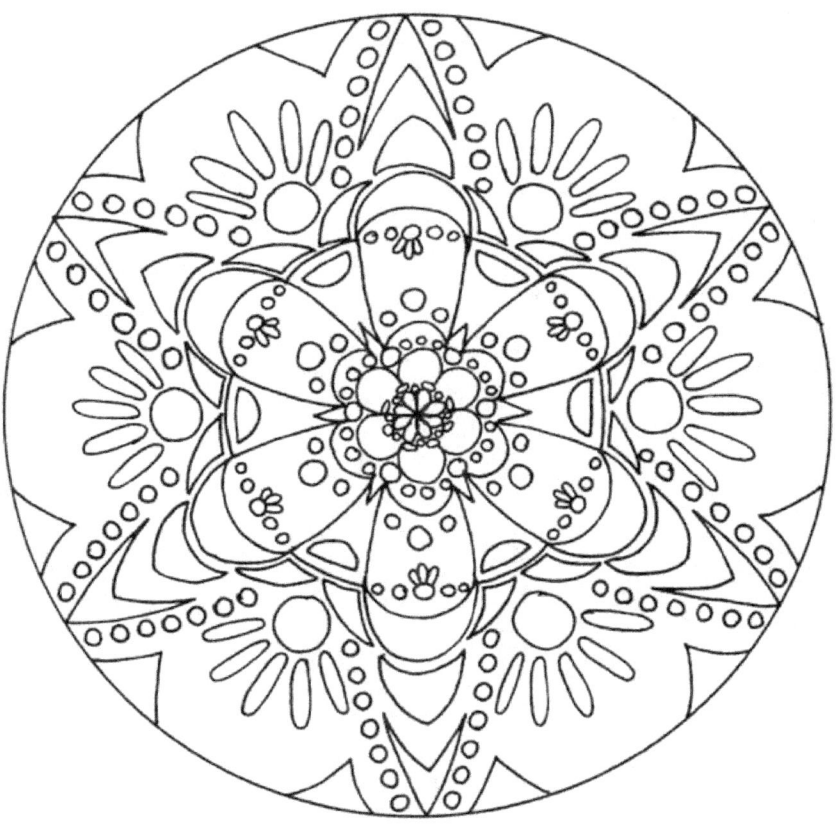

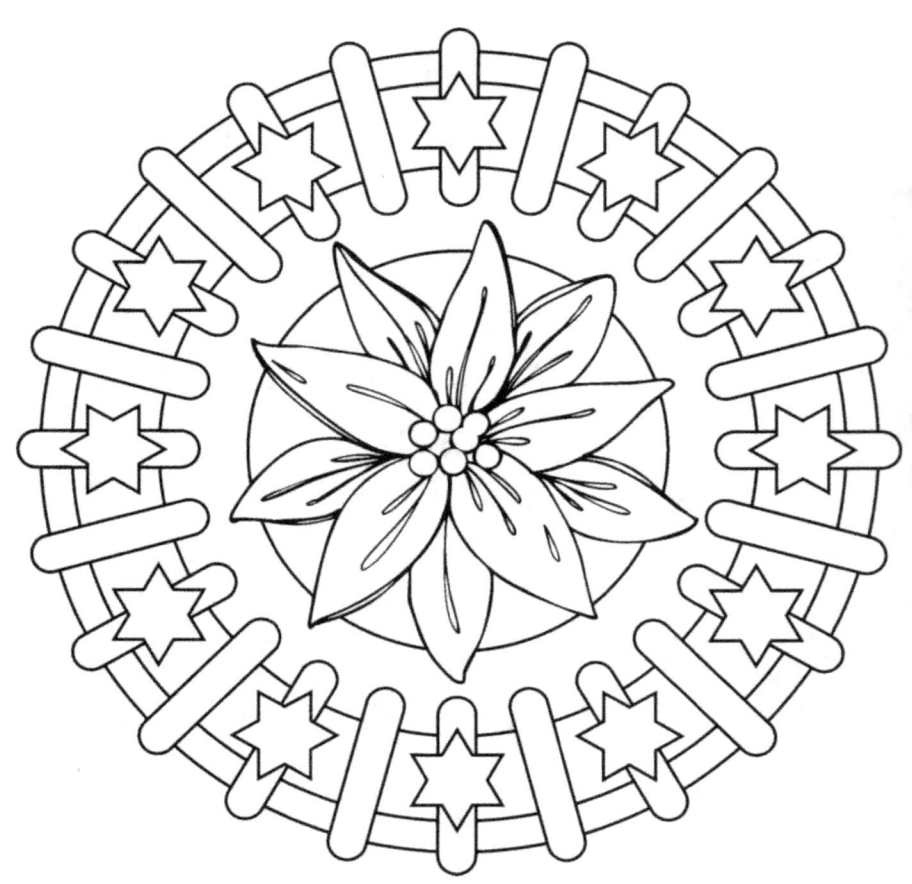

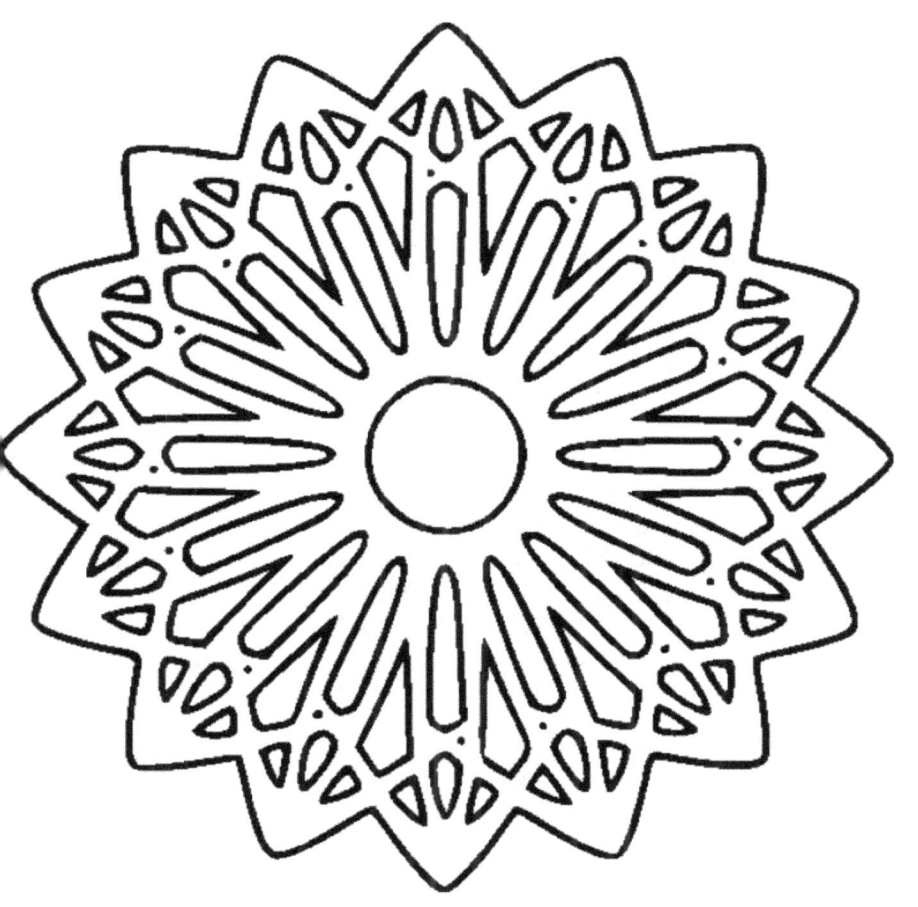

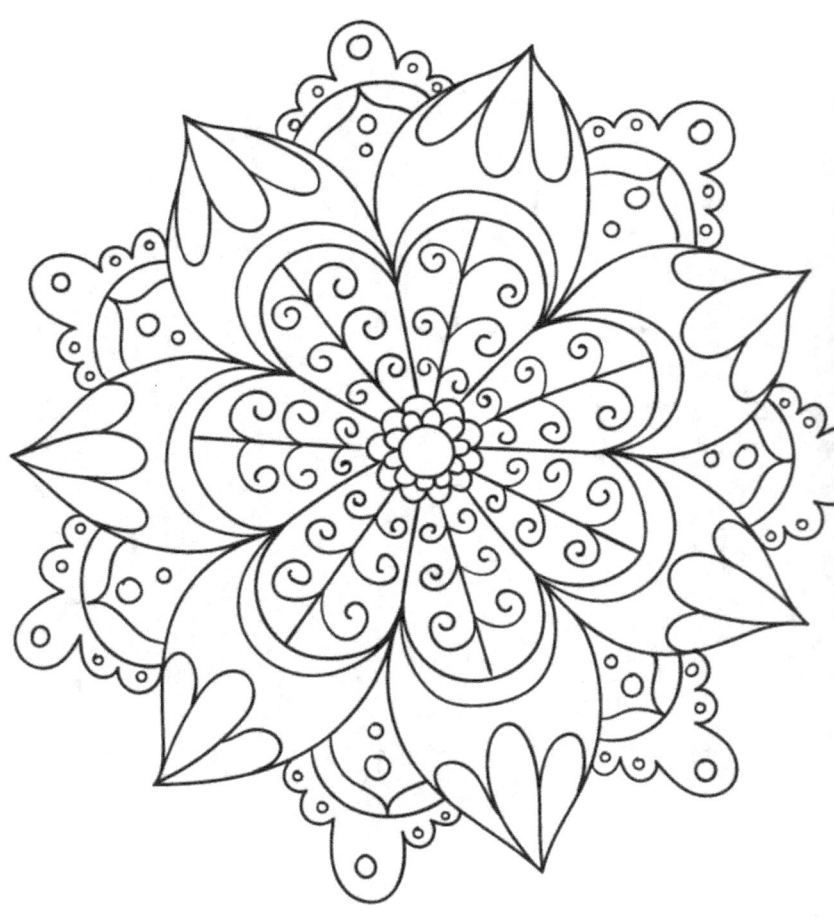

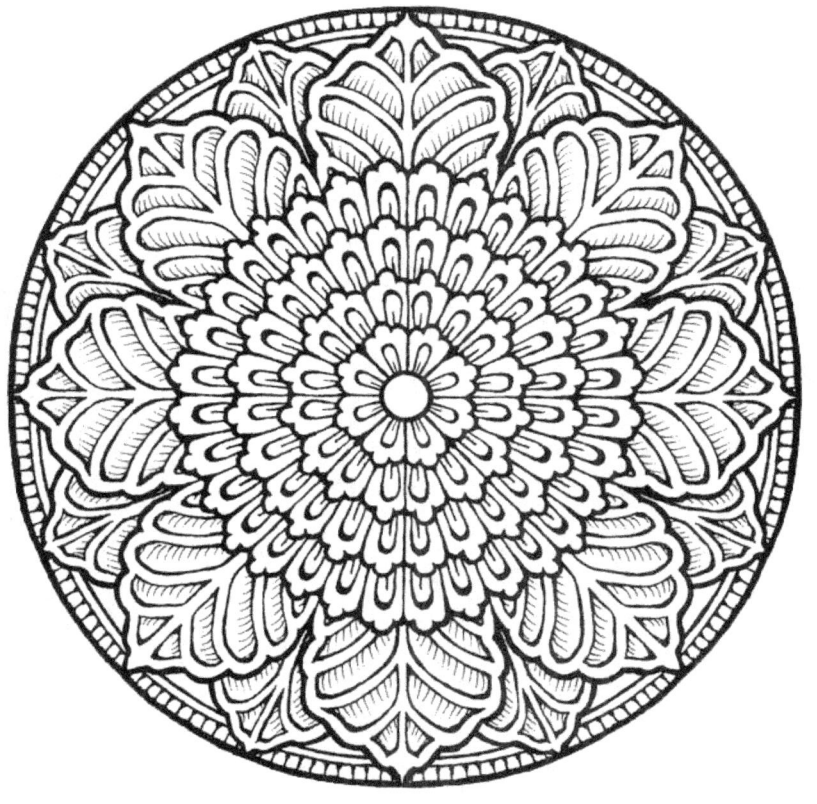

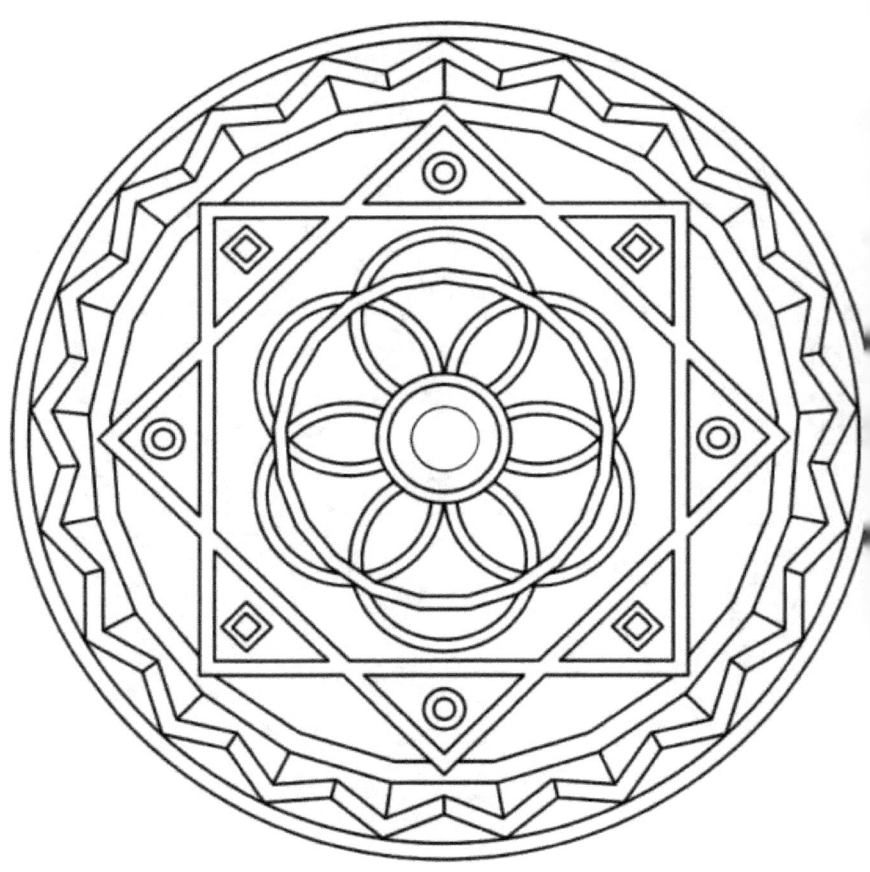

ABOUT THE AUTHOR

Lamees A. is a prolific, inspirational writer and artist.
For other books by Lamees A. please visit
http://amzn.to/1WIsY36

Visit http://www.lameesauthor.com/
And get free Adult Coloring Books.